tredition

tredition was established in 2006 by Sandra Latusseck and Soenke Schulz. Based in Hamburg, Germany, tredition offers publishing solutions to authors and publishing houses, combined with worldwide distribution of printed and digital book content. tredition is uniquely positioned to enable authors and publishing houses to create books on their own terms and without conventional manufacturing risks.

For more information please visit: www.tredition.com

TREDITION CLASSICS

This book is part of the TREDITION CLASSICS series. The creators of this series are united by passion for literature and driven by the intention of making all public domain books available in printed format again - worldwide. Most TREDITION CLASSICS titles have been out of print and off the bookstore shelves for decades. At tredition we believe that a great book never goes out of style and that its value is eternal. Several mostly non-profit literature projects provide content to tredition. To support their good work, tredition donates a portion of the proceeds from each sold copy. As a reader of a TREDITION CLASSICS book, you support our mission to save many of the amazing works of world literature from oblivion. See all available books at www.tredition.com.

 Project Gutenberg

The content for this book has been graciously provided by Project Gutenberg. Project Gutenberg is a non-profit organization founded by Michael Hart in 1971 at the University of Illinois. The mission of Project Gutenberg is simple: To encourage the creation and distribution of eBooks. Project Gutenberg is the first and largest collection of public domain eBooks.

Apis Mellifica or, The Poison of the Honey-Bee, Considered as a Therapeutic Agent

C. W. Wolf

Imprint

This book is part of TREDITION CLASSICS

Author: C. W. Wolf
Cover design: Buchgut, Berlin – Germany

Publisher: tredition GmbH, Hamburg - Germany
ISBN: 978-3-8472-1323-9

www.tredition.com
www.tredition.de

Copyright:
The content of this book is sourced from the public domain.

The intention of the TREDITION CLASSICS series is to make world literature in the public domain available in printed format. Literary enthusiasts and organizations, such as Project Gutenberg, worldwide have scanned and digitally edited the original texts. tredition has subsequently formatted and redesigned the content into a modern reading layout. Therefore, we cannot guarantee the exact reproduction of the original format of a particular historic edition. Please also note that no modifications have been made to the spelling, therefore it may differ from the orthography used today.

Apis Mellifica;

or,

THE POISON OF THE HONEY-BEE.

Considered as a Therapeutic Agent.

BY C. W. WOLF, M.D.,

Ex-District Physician in Berlin.

PHILADELPHIA:
PUBLISHED AND FOR SALE BY
WILLIAM RADDE, 635 ARCH STREET.
1858.

APIS MELLIFICA;
OR,
THE POISON OF THE HONEY-BEE,
Considered as a Therapeutic Agent.

BY C. W. WOLF, M.D.,
Ex-District Physician in Berlin.

PUBLISHED AND FOR SALE BY

WILLIAM RADDE, 635 ARCH STREET.
1858.

PREFACE.

Every physician who has spent years of an active life in prescribing for large numbers of patients, is morally bound to publish his experience to the world, provided he is satisfied, in his interior conscience, that such a publication might be useful to the general interests of humanity.

In offering the following essay to my readers, I simply desire to fulfil an obligation recognised as valid by the inner sense. This essay contains every thing that an experience of forty years in the conscientious and philanthropic exercise of my profession has sanctioned and confirmed as truth. Nor have I adopted a single fact, suggested by my own observation, as correct, without contrasting it with the most approved records of medicine. To every true friend of man, and more particularly to every physician who considers the business of healing disease as the highest [4] office of medical art, I offer this essay for further trial and examination. May the statements expressed in it either be confirmed or else corrected and improved by those who excel in more thorough knowledge and ability.

The Author.

Berlin, Oct., 1857.

[5]

APIS MELLIFICA.

"The bee helps to heal all thy internal and external maladies, and is the best little friend whom man possesses in this world."—More in Cotton's *Book of the Bee*, p. 138.

Since Hahnemann's successful attempt to develop the medicinal nature of Aconite, no other discovery has been made in the domain of practical medicine, as comprehensive and universally useful as the discovery of the medicinal virtues of the poison of the bee. It is of the utmost importance to the interests of humanity to become as intimately acquainted with the efficacy of this poison as possible. It is the object of these papers to contribute my mite to this work.

As soon as Dr. Hering had published the provings of the bee poison, in his "American Provings," I at once submitted them to the test of experience in an extensive practice. I prepared the drug which I used for this purpose, by pouring half an ounce of alcohol on five living bees, and shaking them during the space of eight days, three times a-day, with one hundred vigorous strokes of the arm. From this preparation, which I used as the mother-tincture, I obtained attenuations up to the thirties centesimal scale. So far, the effects which I have [6] obtained with this preparation, have been uniformly satisfactory. It has seemed to me that the lower potencies lose in power as they are kept for a longer period; hence, I consider it safer to prepare them fresh every year. As a general rule, I have found either the third or the thirtieth potency, sufficient.

Day after day I have obtained more satisfactory results, and now I look upon Apis mellifica as the greatest polychrest, next to Aconite, which we possess.

The introduction of this poison to the medical profession, will be looked upon as the most brilliant merit of one of the most deserving apostles of homœopathy, and will secure immortality to the honored name of Constantine Hering. The following statements will show how far this faith of a grateful heart is founded upon facts:

Apis mellifica is the most satisfactory remedy for acute hydrocephalus of children.

The more acute and dangerous the attack, the more readily will it yield to the action of Apis. Sudden convulsions, followed by general fever, loss of consciousness, delirium, sopor while the child is lying in bed, interrupted more or less by sudden cries; boring of the head into the pillow, with copious sweat about the head, having the odor of musk; inability to hold the head erect; squinting of one or both eyes; dilatation of the pupils; gritting of the teeth; protrusion of the tongue; desire to vomit; nausea, retching and vomiting; collapse of the abdominal walls; scanty urine, which is [7] sometimes milky; costiveness; trembling of the limbs; occasional twitching of the limbs on one side of the body, and apparent paralysis of those of the other side; painful turning inwards of the big toes, extorting cries from the patient; accelerated pulse, which soon becomes slower, irregular, intermittent and rather hard; these symptoms inform us that life is in danger, the more so the more numerous they are grouped together.

In comparing with these symptoms the following symptoms from Hering's American Provings, Part I., 3d Num., p. 294: "40, 41, muttering during sleep; muttering and delirium during sleep; 83, 84, he had lost all consciousness of the things around him; he sank into a state of insensibility; 140, 144, sense of weight and fulness in the fore part of the head; heaviness and fulness in the vertex; dull pain in the occiput, aggravated by shaking the head; pressure, fulness and heaviness in the occiput; 170, her whole brain feels tired, as if gone to sleep; tingling; she experiences the same sensation in both arms, especially in the left, and from the left knee down to the foot; 175, 176, sensation as if the head were too large; swelling of the head; 391, when biting the teeth together, swallowing; after gaping or at other times, a sort of gritting the teeth; only a single, involuntary jerk frequently repeated; 501, nausea and vomiting; 506, nausea, as if one would vomit, with fainting; 512, vomiting of the ingesta; 619, retention of stool; 640, retention of urine; 665, scanty and dark-colored urine; 980, 984, 985, trembling, convulsions, starting during sleep as if [8] in affright; 1020, sudden weakness, compelling him to lie down; he lost all recollection; 1032, great desire for sleep, he felt extremely drowsy." If we compare these effects of Apis to the above-mentioned symptoms of hydrocephalus, we shall find the homœopathicity of Apis to this disease more than superficially indicated. If we consider, moreover, that the known effects of Apis show that it possesses the power of exciting inflammatory irritation and œdematous swellings, we are justified, by our law of similarity, in expecting curative results from the use of Apis in all such diseases.

The experiments which I have instituted for the last four years, have convinced me of the correctness of this observation. Whenever I had an opportunity of giving Apis at the commencement of the diseases, it would produce within twelve to twenty-four hours quiet sleep; general perspiration, affording relief; the feverish and nervous symptoms, together with the delirium, would disappear from hour to hour, and on waking, the little patient's consciousness was lucid, the appetite good and recovery fully established. This is a triumph of art which inspires us with admiration for our science. Less surprising, but equally certain, is the relief, if Apis is given after the disease has lasted for some time. In such a case, the medicine first excites a combat between the morbific force and the conservative reaction. The greater the hostile force, the longer the struggle between momentary improvement and aggravation of the symptoms; it may sometimes continue for one, two, or three days. It [9] is not until now, that a progressive and permanent improvement sets in. The desire to vomit is gone; the twitching, trembling, and the struggle, generally diminish from hour to hour; consciousness returns; the squinting and the dilatation of the pupils abate; gritting of the teeth and protrusion of the tongue cease; the position and movements of the head and limbs become more natural; the pulse becomes more regular; its slowness yields to a more normal frequency; the feverish heat terminates in sweat which affords great relief, and the retention of stool and urine is succeeded by a more copious action of both the bowels and bladder. The natural appetite returns; the reproductive process is restored; sleep is quiet and refreshing, and recovery is perfectly established in an incredibly short period. A cure of this kind generally requires five, seven, eleven, and fourteen days. This result is so favorable, that those who have not witnessed it, or who are too ignorant and egotistical to investigate the facts, may reject it as incredible.

Such brilliant results are obtained by means of a single drop of Apis, third attenuation. I mix a drop with seven tablespoonfuls of water, and give a dessert-spoonful every hour, or every two or three hours; the more acute the attack, the more frequently the dose is repeated; this method generally suffices to effect a cure more or less rapidly. As long as the improvement progresses satisfactorily, all we have to do is to let the medicine act without interfering. If the improvement is arrested, or the patient gets worse, which sometimes happens in the more intense grades of this malady, the best course [10] is to give a globule of Apis 30, and to watch the result for some twenty-four hours. After the lapse of this period the improvement will either have resumed its course, or else it will continue unsatisfactory. In the latter case we should give another dose of the above-mentioned solution of Apis 3. Not unfrequently I have met with patients upon whom Apis acts too powerfully, causing pains in the bowels, interminable diarrhœa, of a dysenteric character, extreme prostration and a sense of fainting. In such cases the tumultuous action of Apis is mitigated, and the continued use of this drug, rendered possible by giving Apis in alternation with Aconite in water, every hour or two hours.

Except such cases, I have never been obliged to resort to other accessory means.

Apis is no less efficacious against the higher grades of ophthalmia.

It is particularly rheumatic, catarrhal, erysipelatous, and œdematous ophthalmia, which is most rapidly, easily, and safely cured by Apis, no matter what part of the eye may be the seat of the disease.

The symptoms 188-307 distinctly point to the curative virtues of Apis in ophthalmia: "Sensitiveness to light, with headache, redness of the eyes; he keeps his eyes closed, light is intolerable, the eyes are painful and feel sore and irritated if he uses them; weakness of sight, with feeling of fullness in the eyes; twitching of the left eyeball; feeling of heaviness in the eyelids and eyes; aching, sore-pressing, tensive, shooting, boring, stinging, burning pains in and around the eyes, and above the eyes in [11] the forehead; redness of the eyes and lids; secretion of mucus and agglutination of the lids; the lids are swollen, dark-red, everted; the conjunctiva is reddened, full of dark blood-vessels which gradually lose themselves in the cornea; the cornea is obscured, smoky, showing a few little ulcers here and there; profuse lachrymation; stinging itching in the left eye, in the lids and around the eye; sensation of a quantity of mucus in the left eye; sensation of a foreign little body in the eye; soreness of the canthi; styes; œdema of the lids; erysipelatous inflammation of the lids."

I have found the correctness of these observations uniformly confirmed by the most satisfactory cures of such affections. I use the medicine in the same manner as for acute hydrocephalus. In some cases I found the eye so sensitive to the action of Apis, that an exceedingly violent aggravation of the inflammatory symptoms ensued, which might have proved dangerous to the preservation of such a delicate organ as the eye. Inasmuch as it is impossible to determine beforehand the degree of sensitiveness, I obviate all danger by exhibiting Apis in alternation with Aconite in the manner indicated for hydrocephalus. By means of this alternate exhibition of two drugs, we not only prevent every aggravating primary effect, but we at the same time act in accordance with the important law, that, in order to secure the effective and undisturbed repetition of a drug, we have first to interrupt its action by some appropriate intermediate remedy. All repetitions should cease as soon as a [12] general improvement sets in; if the medicine is continued beyond the point where the organism is saturated with the drug, it acts as a hostile agent, not as a curative remedy. This important point is known by the fact, that the improvement which had already commenced, seems to remain stationary; the patient experiences a distressing urging to stool, a burning diarrhœa sets in, and a disproportionate feeling of malaise develops itself. Under these circumstances, a globule of Apis 30 will quiet the patient, and the action of the drug will achieve the cure without any further difficulty, and without much loss of time, unless psora, sycosis, syphilis, or vaccine-virus prevail in the organism, or sulphur, iodine or mercury had been previously given in large doses. In the presence of such complications Apis will prove ineffectual until they have been removed by some specific antidote. After having made a most careful diagnosis, a single dose of the highest potency of the specific remedy be given, and be allowed to act as long as a trace of improvement is still perceptible. As soon as the improvement ceases, or an aggravation of the symptoms sets in, Apis is in its place and will act most satisfactorily. We then give Apis 3 in water, as mentioned above, with the most satisfactory success.

Apis is the most appropriate remedy for inflammation of the tongue, mouth, and throat.

The following symptoms may be looked upon as striking curative indications: 378-380, 383, 384, 399, 400, 405, 406, 409, 410, 413, 419, 436, 437, [13] 439, 443, 444, 449, 455, 458, 459, 463, 470, 471: "Burning of the lips; the upper lip is swollen to such a degree that the inside seems turned outside; swelling of the lips and tongue; swelling of the upper lip, it becomes hot and red, almost brown; dark streaks along the vermilion border, particularly on the upper lip, rough, cracked, peeling off; violent pains spreading through the gums, the gums bleed readily; the tongue feels as if burnt; tongue and palate are sore; raw feeling, burning, blisters along the margin of the tongue, very painful, stinging; at the tip of the tongue a row of small vesicles which cause a pain as if sore and raw; dry tongue; the inner cheeks look red and fiery, with painful sensitiveness; inflammation of the tongue; inflammation and swelling of the palate; burning, stinging sensation in the mouth and throat; pressure in the fauces as of a foreign body; ptyalism; copious accumulation of a soapy mucus in the mouth and throat; dryness and heat in the throat; inability to swallow a drop, with swelling of the tongue; sensation of gnawing and contraction in the throat, increasing after four hours so as to render deglutition difficult; sensation of fulness, constriction and suffocation in the throat; deglutition painful and impeded, stinging pains during deglutition; swelling and redness of the tonsils, impeding deglutition; angina faucium; chilliness followed by heat; violent pain in the temples; redness and swelling of the tonsils; uvula and fauces, painful and impeded deglutition, and stinging pains when attempting to swallow." [14]

The more frequently we make use of Apis in the treatment of these very common forms of angina, and of the inflammation of the salivary glands, which are so closely connected with the other parts of the throat, the more we become convinced by the most striking success, that this drug is by far the speediest, safest and easiest remedy which we possess for the treatment of these exceedingly common and yet so very distressing affections. Not only in common affections of this sort, but also in the most acute and dangerous forms of angina faucium, will Apis be found efficient; even where these affections are hereditary, or have become habitual, and generally terminate in suppuration, Apis will still afford help. In these affections likewise Apis acts most promptly and efficiently, if given in alternation with Aconite, both remedies in the third dilution, a few drops dissolved in twelve tablespoonfuls of water, in alternate hourly doses. After taking a few doses, the patient begins to feel relieved, enjoys a quiet sleep, and the resolution of the inflammation takes place, accompanied by the breaking out of a general perspiration. If there should be a natural tendency to suppuration, this treatment will hasten it from hour to hour, and after the pus is discharged, a cure will soon be accomplished. In the most inveterate cases, which had been previously treated in a different manner, the same curative process takes place gradually; first one outbreak of the disease is hushed; next, if another portion of the throat becomes inflamed, this inflammation is controlled, [15] and this proceeding is continued with an increasingly rapid success and a continued abatement of all sufferings, until, finally, a perfect recovery is obtained, even under these disadvantageous circumstances.

Apis is not sufficient to prevent the recurrence of such inflammatory attacks; this object has to be accomplished by means of the appropriate antidotal specific.

Apis becomes an exceedingly useful remedy in consequence of the specific power which it possesses over the whole internal mucous membrane and its appendages.

It is particularly the mucous membrane of the alimentary canal upon which Apis has a striking influence. It excites an inflammatory irritation, which not only disturbs the secretion of mucus, but also disintegrates the intestinal juices so essential to the process of sanguification, thus disqualifying the blood from properly contributing to the reproduction of the nervous tissue. By thus altering the blood and nerves, these two principal vehicles of vitality, it develops a group of symptoms which is exceedingly similar to our abdominal typhus that seems to have become stationary among us for the last twenty years. This similarity, in its totality, results from the following symptoms contained in the "American Provings."

"398: troublesome pains in the gums. 400: the gums bleed readily. 402: bitterish taste in the back part of the tongue and in the throat. 405: tongue as if burnt. 406: tongue and palate feel [16] sore. 411: a number of vesicles and small, sore, somewhat red spots at the tip of the tongue and along the left margin of the tongue. 413: dry tongue, the inner cheeks look red, fiery, are painfully sensitive. 416: burning from the tongue down the œsophagus, as far as the stomach, eructations every four or five minutes, with flow of tasteless water in the mouth; eructations became worse after drinking water, she almost felt as if choked. 420: swelling of the tongue, the tongue is dry, shining, yellowish. 421: tenacious saliva adhering to the tongue. 424: tongue dry and white. 427: feeling of dryness in the mouth and throat. 441: fetid breath, with gastritis. 445: quantity of thick, tenacious mucus deep in the throat, obliging him to hawk. 447: tenacious, frothy saliva. 450: dryness in the throat, without thirst. 452: loathing, as if out of the throat. 459: sense of fulness, constriction and choking in the throat. 474: loss of taste. 475: complete loss of appetite. 488: no thirst, with heat. 492: very thirsty when waking at night, after diarrhœa. 495: eructations tasting of white of eggs. 501: nausea and vomiting. 504: fainting sort of nausea from the short ribs across the whole abdomen. 512: vomiting of the ingesta. 513: vomiting of bile. 516: vomiting and diarrhœa. 517: nausea, vomiting of the ingesta, and diarrhœa; repeated vomiting, first of bile, afterwards a thin, watery fluid, having a very bitter taste, with violent pains across the abdomen. 518 to 525: oppression, pressing, creeping, drawing and gnawing, pricking, soreness, heat and burning in the stomach. [17] 528: painful sensitiveness in the pit of the stomach, with burning, like heartburn, with bilious diarrhœa, rather greenish, and almost painless. 530: violent pain and sensitiveness in the region of the stomach and epigastrium, with vomiting, coated tongue, fetid breath, costiveness, and sleep disturbed by muttering and dreams, with frequent, wiry pulse. 533: sense of numbness under the right ribs. 532: sense of compression, squeezing, bruising, under the ribs, worse on the left side. 535: violent burning pains under the short ribs on both sides, worst and most permanent on the left side, *where the pain is felt for weeks, preventing sleep.* 543: rumbling in the abdomen, with violent urging to stool. 545: nausea in the abdomen, has to lie down. 546: weight in the abdomen. 547: dull pain in the bowels. 552: occasional attacks of colic, with a feverish, tremulous sensation. 553: violent, cutting pains in the abdomen. 555: slowly pulsating, boring pain above the left crest of the ilium, relieved by eructations. 556: pain in the abdomen, from the hips to the umbilical region. 560: soreness and pressure in the lower abdomen. 563: *feeling of soreness, burning and numbness below and on the side of the right hip, deep-seated.* 566: the inner abdomen feels sore and as if excoriated, painful when pressed upon. 567: feeling as if the bowels had been squeezed, with tenesmus during stool. 576: fulness and sense of distension in the abdomen, as if bloated. 589: frequent urging to stool, with pain in the anus on account of the frequent pressing. 590: violent tenesmus. 593: several thin, yellow evacuations, [18] accompanied by excessive prostration; the stools set in at every motion of the body, as if the anus were wide open. 598: copious discharges of dark brown, green and whitish excrements. 599: dysenteric stools. 608: blood and mucus with stool. 611 and 612: painful and also painless diarrhœa, especially in the morning. 617: retention of stool for one week. 646: disagreeable sensation in the bladder, with pressing downwards in the region of the sphincter, and frequent urging, so that he voids urine frequently in the day-time, and ten or twelve times at night; burning and cutting during urination. 668: the urine is dark colored. 730: hoarseness and distress of breathing. 733: roughness and sensitiveness in the larynx. 738: violent cough, especially after lying down and sleeping. 754: hurried and difficult breathing, with heat and headache. 803: sense of soreness, lameness, bruised and contusive feeling in the chest. 812: trembling and pressure in the chest, with embarrassed breathing. 818: pulse scarcely perceptible. 822: pulse accelerated. 833: swelling of the cervical glands on the injured side. 968: extreme sensitiveness of the whole body to contact, every hair is painful when touched. 971: excessive nervousness. 979: general lassitude, with trembling. 994: in the afternoon he becomes extremely restless and exhausted. 1011: paroxysms of great weakness. 1021: sudden weakness, he had to lie down, and lost his senses. 1025: complete loss of recollection, with vomiting, desire for sleep and rest, slow beating of the heart and scarcely perceptible pulse. 1032: excessive drowsiness. [19] 1039: starting during sleep, as if in affright, with some cough. 1046: sleeplessness. 1047: restless sleep, frequent waking and constant *dreaming*. 1064: chattering during sleep (in the case of a child). 1081: chilly every afternoon at three or four o'clock, she feels a shivering, worse during warmth; chilly creepings across the back, the hands feel numb; an hour after, feverish heat, with rough cough, hot cheeks and hands, no thirst; these symptoms pass off gradually, but she feels heavy and prostrated. 1089: chill after a heat of thirty-six hours. 1090: sudden chilliness, afterwards heat and sweat. 1124: alternate sweat and dry skin. 1198: thick urticaria, itching a great deal (very soon). 1224: swelling and erysipelatous redness. 54: unable to concentrate his thoughts. 57: dulness of the head, it feels compressed. 62: vertigo and weakness. 79: dizziness."

Whosoever compares the totality of these effects of Apis to the symptoms of the prevailing abdominal typhus, will admit that Apis is homœopathic to this disease. He will even admit that this homœopathicity of Apis to abdominal typhus extends to the minute particulars of the disease *in their totality*. Even the course which Apis pursues, in developing its effects in the organism, is similar to the progressive development of typhus. Any one who has witnessed, as I have, the course which this disease pursues, will admit that mucous membrane of the alimentary canal is first affected by the disease, in the same manner as Apis affects it; that this irritation of the mucous membrane is followed by [20] gastric catarrhal symptoms, which are speedily succeeded by symptoms of disintegration of the animal fluids and typhoid phenomena; that the gastric irritation is generally characterized by boils, urticaria, erysipelas of the skin, and the nervous irritation by symptoms of abdominal typhus; that the internal and external development of the disease is determined by a striking sympathetic derangement of the organic functions of the liver, and still more of the spleen, and likewise by a more striking prominence of the intermittent type of the fever; and that all these varied disturbances finally culminate in abdominal typhus.

Owing to this remarkable similarity, Apis will effect striking cures of all these different derangements.

If, after more or less distinctly felt premonitory symptoms — after a sudden cold, excessive exertions, prostrating emotions or enjoyments — a more or less violent fever is developed, accompanied by dulness and painfulness of the head, retching and vomiting, distention and sensitiveness of the pit of the stomach, and soon after of the whole abdomen, with urging diarrhœa, pappy and foul taste in the mouth, loss of appetite and thirst, feeling of dryness in the mouth and throat, tongue sore, as if burnt and swollen, with antagonistic change of symptoms, suspicious and extraordinary prostration, and feeling of fainting; a few spoonfuls of the above-mentioned solution of Apis 3, will afford such speedy relief, that it may seem incredible to those who have not witnessed it. The nausea, the vomiting, the diarrhœa, [21] and the painfulness of the abdomen, disappear; quiet sleep sets in, with general perspiration, which terminates the fever, and affords great relief; after waking, the patient is comforted by the internal sensation of returning health; a natural appetite is again felt, the strength returns, and in a few days the healthy look of the tongue and buccal cavity shows that the mucous membrane of the stomach and bowels has recovered its normal quality. The longer help is deferred, the longer time the morbid process has had in making its inroads upon the system, the more frequently will it be necessary to repeat the medicine, until a cure is achieved.

The same good result is perceived, if the morbid process is accompanied by furuncles, urticaria, erysipelas—the latter principally on the head and in the face, less frequently upon the extremities, and inclining to shift from one place to another. Such a combination of symptoms not only shows a higher degree of intensity of the disease, but also shows that the organism is still capable of battling against the internal disease, by compelling it to leave the interior tissue, and to develop itself externally. It is the first business of the physician to support the organism in this tendency, and to guard the brain and bowels from every destructive relapse. Apis, employed as above, accomplishes this result more speedily than any other drug. Of course, a few days are required for this purpose, although the rules of using the drug and the course of treatment are the same.

The same observation applies to the not unfrequent [22] complication with organic disease of the spleen and consequent dropsy. Apis, used in the same manner, effects, in as short a period as the intensity of the symptoms will permit, a mitigation and gradual disappearance of the painfulness of the spleen, restores the normal action of the spleen more and more, and neutralises the tendency to dropsical effusion at the same time as it expels the accumulated fluid by increasing the secretions from the bladder and bowels, and the cutaneous exhalation.

If the liver is organically diseased, Apis is no longer sufficient. In such a case, the action of the liver has first to be restored to its normal standard. In dropsical diseases, I have effected this result most frequently, for years past, by means of Carduus mariæ, less frequently by Quassia, still less frequently by Nux vomica, and only in a few cases by Chelidonium: according as one or the other of these agents seemed indicated by the epidemic character of the disease. In all non-malignant cases, if the medicine was permitted to act in time, the whole disease was often cut short by the use of these drugs, and the development of typhoid symptoms prevented. Not, however, in all more inveterate cases, where the prevailing character of the disease, by its more penetrating action upon the tissues, induced a slower and more threatening course of development. As soon as the pains in the right hypochondrium had disappeared, the bilious quality of the fæces had been restored, and the urine had become lighter colored, but the fever still continued, tongue, throat, pit of the stomach and abdomen had [23] become more sensitive; the head duller and tighter, and the prostration more overpowering. In such a case, Apis, prepared as above, became indispensable, in order to remove all danger to life. Its curative action soon became manifest in two different ways.

If the reactive force of the organism was still sufficient, the medicine succeeded very speedily in preventing the supervention of the typhoid stage, in changing the fever-type from a remittent or even continuous to an intermittent type, during which the convalescence of the patient, aided by a suitable diet, was more and more firmly established and generally completely secured after the lapse of a week.

If the typhoid stage could not be prevented and set in with the following symptoms: the patient lies on his bed in a state of apathy, with loss of recollection, sopor, muttering delirium, hardness of hearing, inability to protrude the tongue or to articulate; dry, cracked, sore, blistered, ulcerated tongue; difficult deglutition; painful distention of the abdomen, which is sensitive to contact or pressure; retention of stool, or else frequent, painful, foul, bloody, involuntary diarrhœa; fermentous urine, which is sometimes discharged involuntarily; the skin is at times and partially dry, burning, at times and partially clammy, cool; trembling and twitching of the limbs; white miliaria on the chest and abdomen; extreme debility, with settling towards the foot-end of the bed; changing pulse, which is at times slow, at others accelerated, feeble, intermittent: in such a case [24] Apis requires more time to heal the mucous membrane of the alimentary canal; to restore the normal action of the bowels; to regulate the digestive functions; to procure quiet and refreshing sleep, and to gradually effect a complete restoration of health. If the mucous membrane of the respiratory organs was invaded by the morbid process, the cure was nevertheless completed as soon as the mucous lining of the intestinal canal was restored to its natural condition.

So far, the only obstacle to a cure which I have witnessed, has been tuberculosis of the chest or abdominal viscera, or of both at the same time, and still more the vaccine-virus; likewise a tendency to paralysis in persons who were otherwise morbidly affected. Tuberculosis has often been combated by a single dose of a high potence of Sulphur between the doses of Apis, no Apis being given after the Sulphur, as long as the course of the typhoid symptoms would render it safe to postpone this medicine. I have found it much more difficult to conquer the vaccine-poison, *which I have become satisfied by years of observation, constitutes the most universal and most powerful generator of the typhus which is prevailing in our age and which seems unwilling to leave us.* Tartar emetic proves in this, as in other cases, its antidotal power against the vaccine-virus; but under no circumstances is more caution required in the use of tartar emetic than in typhus, where the vaccine-virus seeks to develop its characteristic pustules with a tendency inherent in each pustule to terminate in the destruction [25] of the mucous membrane. It may seem hazardous to add to this combination of destructive forces another similarly-acting element; but a careful consideration of the circumstances of the case will justify such a proceeding, although death may be the inevitable result of the morbid process. Experience has satisfied me that the alternate use of tartar emetic and Apis, a drop of the third potency of each, every three, six or twelve hours, according as the symptoms are more or less violent, or, in very sensitive organisms, in tablespoonful doses of a watery solution of a drop, will accomplish all that can be expected; for these two drugs, thus administered, seem to compensate or complete each other. I am unable to say how far this proceeding requires to be modified in particular cases; all I desire to do, is to submit this important subject to my colleagues for further inquiry and trial.

If a tendency to paralysis prevails, the danger is less threatening, although equally momentous. In such cases I use Apis and Moschus in alternation, although I am unable to assert, on account of deficient experience, that this treatment will always prove satisfactory. Such cases hardly ever arise under homœopathic treatment; and if they come to us out of the hands of allœopathic practitioners, they generally prove incurable.

If these three obstacles to a cure appear combined, I have never found it possible to effect any thing. All that I have found it possible to do, has been to prevent such a dreadful combination by [26] carefully attending to my patients in previous diseases.

Sometimes in typhus, the affection of the spleen shows itself again, even after recovery has fairly set in; the intermittent type again breaks forth, and recovery finally takes place, as the intermissions become more and more distinct and lengthened. As long as the intermittent type continues, Apis has to be given; the action of the spleen becomes more and more normal, the fever paroxysms become shorter and less marked, and the restoration of health is effected without any more treatment than a single dose of Apis 30, one globule, which is permitted to act until the patient is well.

Observations of this kind, which I have made under the most diversified circumstances, have taught me that Apis is *the most sovereign remedy for all those morbid processes which we designate as* INTERMITTENT FEVER.

The following symptoms indicate the homœopathicity of Apis to intermittent fever:

"1081: every afternoon about three or four o'clock she feels chilly, shivering, worse in warmth; a chilly creeping along the back, the hands seem dead; in about an hour she feels feverish and hot, with rough cough, hot hands and cheeks, without thirst; these symptoms pass off gradually, after which she feels heavy and prostrate. 1088: chilliness all over, recurring periodically, with an undulating sensation. 1089: chill after a heat of thirty-six hours. 1090: sudden chilliness, followed by heat and sweat. 499: loathing, with chilliness and [27] coldness of the limbs. 534: pains on the left side, below the last ribs. 535: violent burning pain below the short ribs, on both sides, worst and most permanent on the left side, where it continues for weeks, preventing sleep. 577: enlargement of the abdomen, with swelling of the feet, scanty urine."

The provings of Apis show that this drug affects every portion of the nervous system—the cerebral, spinal and ganglionic nerves—and the process of sanguification, in the same general and characteristic manner as is the case in fever and ague.

In comparing the symptoms of Apis with those of any other known drug, there is no medicine that bears as close an affinity to fever and ague as Apis. Howsoever useful other remedies may have proved, in the treatment of fever and ague, they are only homœopathic to isolated conditions, in comparison with Apis. In practice, it was often found very difficult, even for the most experienced physician, to decide in which of these exceptional cases the specifically homœopathic agent should have been employed. Sometimes no properly homœopathic remedy could be found, in which case the treatment had to be conducted in a round-about way.

All these difficulties have been effectually removed by Apis, and the treatment of intermittent fever may henceforth be said to constitute one of the most certain and positive achievements of the homœopathic domain. For the last three years, during which period I have experimented with Apis, I have not come across a single case of intermittent fever that did not yield satisfactorily to [28] Apis. I have treated a pretty fair share of obstinate and complicated cases of this disease, and have, therefore, had an opportunity of testing the curative virtues of Apis in a satisfactory manner. Here are the results of my observations:

Apis is the natural remedy for the pathological process which is characterized by periodical paroxysms of chill, heat and sweat; the other morbid symptoms being common to this process, as they are to all other diseases.

All the symptoms which have hitherto been observed in intermittent fever, will be found, with striking similarity, among the provings of Apis. For a confirmation of this statement, we refer to Hering's American Provings, and to Bœnninghausen's Essay on Intermittent Fevers.

In making use of Apis in every form of intermittent fever, we not only act in strict accordance with the homœopathic law generally, but we fulfil all the requirements of the individualizing method. Apis is the universal remedy in intermittent fevers, for which every homœopathic physician has been longing, and which pure experiments, conducted according to the rules of homœopathy, have revealed to us; — another shining light on the sublime path of the healing artist!

The beneficent action of Apis, in intermittent fever, is still increased by the fact that it prevents the supervention of typhus, disorganizations of the spleen, dropsy, china-cachexia. In using Apis from the commencement, all such consequences are avoided, and if they should have been induced by [29] different treatment, Apis removes them as speedily as possible.

In all lighter cases, it is sufficient to give a drop of Apis 3, morning and evening, during the apyrexia, and to continue this treatment until the attacks cease; very often no other paroxysm sets in after the first dose; there are scarcely ever more than two or three paroxysms. In a few days the cure is accomplished, provided the action of the medicine is not disturbed.

In more obstinate cases, which had been coming on for a longer period, or had been caused by more noxious influences, had lasted longer, had invaded the organism with more intensity, or where the paroxysms last longer and the intermissions are shorter, or where two paroxysms occur in succession, or the life of the organism is endangered by some cause or other, — the organism has to be saturated with the medicine in the shortest possible period, in order to ensure victory to the curative agent. Under these circumstances, we prepare a solution of from two to four drops of the third potency in twelve tablespoonfuls of water, shake it well in a closed bottle, and give a tablespoonful of this solution every hour. If the case should be urgent, we may give a drop of Apis 3, on sugar, every three or six hours. This treatment is to be continued until the patient is decidedly better; after which the medicine should be discontinued. If the improvement is not quite satisfactory, the last dose is continued several times every twelve or twenty-four hours, after which the proper effect will have [30] been obtained. If the progressive improvement of the patient should be attended with distinct morbid symptoms, it would be injurious to continue the repetition of the drug. Nevertheless, a globule of Apis 30 may sometimes hasten the convalescence of the patient, and otherwise afford relief. Signs of reaction, even if more or less violent, should not deceive one. If left to themselves, they are often and speedily followed by a refreshing calm, and cannot be interfered with, as an aggravation of the symptoms, without damaging the case.

These are all the rules which I have so far been able to infer from my use of Apis. Further experience will have to decide whether they apply to all periods, or only to the prevailing type of fever.

I am unable to say whether Apis will prove effectual against epidemic marsh-intermittents, and if so, how the use of it will have to be modified. May it please those, who can shed light on this subject, to communicate their experience!

Two other exceptions to Apis, as a universal febrifuge, have occurred to me in my practice: *The development of fever and ague in poisoned soil, and fever and ague complicated with China-cachexia.*

It is peculiar to intermittent fever to excite the morbid germs which are slumbering in the organism. This is more particularly true in reference to psora. In proportion to universality of the psoric miasm, fever and ague will develop and complicate itself with psoric affections; and it is such complications that give rise to the inveterate [31] character of intermittents and their disorganizing tendency.

In such cases, a cure cannot be effected without some suitable anti-psoric. During the prevailing fever, Natrum muriaticum has proved such an anti-psoric, provided it was used as follows: If the signs of psoric complication became visible at the outset, I gave a pellet of Natrum mur. 30, and awaited the result until after the third paroxysm. If symptoms of improvement had become manifest, no other remedy was given, and the improvement was permitted to progress from day to day. If the signs of psoric complication were obscure at the beginning of the attack, Apis was at once given. If no improvement became visible after the third paroxysm, or if other symptoms developed themselves, this was looked upon as a proof of the existence of psora, and Natrum mur. 30 was given, and no other remedy, until after the third paroxysm. Either the disease had ceased, or it required further treatment. In the latter case, Apis 3 was continued in drop-doses, morning and evening, until the patient was decidedly convalescent. No further medicine was given after this, and the Natrum mur. was permitted to act undisturbed, without a single repetition. Every such repetition is hurtful; it disturbs the curative process, excites an excess of reaction in the organism, exhausts it, and develops artificial derangements, which often mislead the judgment, and induce an uncalled-for and improper application of remedial means. Such repetitions are unnecessary; any one who is acquainted with the [32] action of Natrum mur., will at once perceive that the psora-destroying effect of this agent had not been neutralized by Apis. Recovery becomes more and more completely established, and sometimes terminates in the breaking out of a wide-spread, bright-looking eruption, resembling recent dry itch, and attended with the peculiar itching which always exists in this disease. The complete peeling off of the epidermis shows the true cause of the disease. In a few cases, an itch-eruption of this kind proved contagious, and communicated itself to other persons in the family.

A similar course of treatment was pursued, if some other antipsoric had to be resorted to, according as one or the other of the three miasms seemed to require.

The thoroughness of this treatment of intermittent fevers is proved by the fact, that no relapses ever took place, or that no secondary diseases were ever developed.

If these sequelæ were the consequences of an abuse of Cinchona, and this China-cachexia was the source of subsequent paroxysms of fever, I have, even in such cases, when nothing else would help, seen Apis cure both the fever and the China-cachexia, in most cases which came under my treatment. In the most inveterate cases, which had perhaps been mismanaged in various ways, and where the reactive power of the organism seemed entirely prostrated, I found it necessary to resort to the employment of a most penetrating agent, more particularly the 5000th potency of Natrum muriaticum, which I have so far found the only sufficiently [33] powerful curative influence under the circumstances. The rules of administering this potency are the same as those for the exhibition of the 30th.

Not only does Apis afford help in the affections which habitually and most generally occur among us; it is likewise in curative rapport with the

Typhoid-gastric conditions which develope themselves during the course of an erysipelatous or exanthematous cutaneous affection, more particularly scarlatina, rubeola, measles and urticaria.

The use of Apis in erysipelas is indicated by: "Nos. 168, 169: great anxiety in the head, with swelling of the face; inflammatory swelling and twitching so violent, that an apoplectic attack is dreaded.

175 to 178: sensation as if the head were too large; swelling of the head; sensitiveness to contact on the vertex, forehead; burning, stinging about the head. 292: erysipelatous inflammation of the eyelids. 295: after the most violent pains of the right eye, a bluish, red, whitish swelling of both eyes, which were closed in consequence. 297: swelling under the eyes during erysipelas, as when stung by a bee. 316: red swelling of both ears, with a stinging and burning pain in the swelling, with redness of the face every evening. 356: erysipelas spreading across the face, and proceeding from the eyes. 359: tension in the face, awakening her about one o'clock, the nose was swollen, so were the right eye and cheek, stinging pain when touching the part; under the right eye, and proceeding from the nose, red streaks spread across the cheek, [34] until four o'clock; next day, after midnight, sudden swelling of the upper lip, with heat and burning redness, continuing until morning; on the third night, sudden crawling over the right cheek, with stinging near the nose, after which the cheek and upper lip swelled. 363: face red and hot, with burning and stinging pain, it swells so that he is no longer recognized. 388: pimple in the vermilion border of the lower lip, which he scratches, after which an erysipelatous swelling arises, spreading rapidly over the chin and the lower jaw, and invading the anterior neck and the glands, so that he is unable to move the jaws, as during trismus, or as if the ligaments of the jaws were inflamed; with constant disposition to sleep, the sleep being interrupted by frightful dreams. 706 to 707: swelling of the right half of the labia, with inflammation and violent pain, rapid, hard pulse, diarrhœa consisting of yellow, greenish mucus, in the case of a girl of three years old; deeply-penetrating distress, commencing in the clitoris and spreading to the vagina; the labia minora are swollen, they feel dry and hard, they are covered with a crust; at the commencement urination is painful. 948: burning of the toes, and erysipelatous redness with heat at a circumscribed spot on the foot, the remainder of the foot being cold. 1167, 1168: acute pain and erysipelatous swelling, hard and white in the centre; bright red, elevated, hard swelling of the place where he was stung, and round about a chilly feeling. 1170-1173: red place where he was stung, with swelling and red streaks along the fingers and [35] arm; red streaks along the lymphatic vessels, proceeding from the sting along the middle finger and arm; inflammatory swelling, spreading all around. 1181: throb-

bing in the swelling. 1182: wide-spread cellular inflammation, terminating in resolution. 1224, 1225: swelling and erysipelatous redness; erysipelatous redness of the toes and feet."

If we add to these remarks, that Apis corresponds to gastric and typhoid conditions, as was shown before, with remarkable similarity of symptoms, we find, without doubt, that all known erysipelatous forms of inflammation are covered by the pathogenetic effects of Apis. Hence we may with propriety give Apis in these affections. Practical experience has abundantly confirmed these conclusions. For the last four years, I have cured readily, safely and easily all forms of erysipelas which have come under my notice—œdematous, smooth, vesicular, light or dark colored, seated or wandering, phlegmonous, recent or habitually recurring, of a light or inveterate character, repelled, among individuals of every disposition and age. I have never seen all kinds of pain yield more readily; I have never seen the accompanying fever abate more speedily; I have never arrested the further spread of erysipelas, nor effected a resolution of the inflammation of the cellular tissue, more certainly; nor, if the termination in suppuration was no longer avoidable, have I ever succeeded in effecting the formation of laudable pus, the spontaneous discharge of the pus, the radical healing of the sore without any scar—*how important is all this in erysipelatous [36] inflammation of the mammæ*—with more certainty and thoroughness, than by means of Apis! No remedy possesses equal powers in protecting internal organs from the dangerous inroad of this disease.

I effected all this without any other medicinal aid, or without resorting to an operation. Keeping quiet and dry, and in a uniform temperature, is all that is required, in order to secure the full curative action of Apis. In this disease it is used in the same manner as we have indicated before. If the liver should be very much involved in this disease, we effect a cure still more rapidly, by alternating Aconite with Apis, in case inflammation is present; Carduus mariæ, in case of simple inflammatory irritation, and Hepatin, if disorganizations have already set in. In phlegmonous and suppurative habitual erysipelas, a cure is generally facilitated, if a dose of Sulphur 30 is interpolated, in the manner which we have explained before, in order to neutralize the psoric taint which is here generally present.

According to this experience, in conjunction with the symptoms 706, 707, I believe that Apis will prove a successful prophylactic and curative agent in a disease of children, which terminates fatally in almost every case. I mean erysipelas of new-born infants, which commences at the genital organs, thence spreads over the skin, and terminates in the induration and destruction of this organ. Until now, I have not had an opportunity of verifying the truth of this theoretical conclusion by actual [37] experiments. Hence I content myself with offering this suggestion for further practical trials.

The American Provings likewise show that Apis may be of great use in scarlatina.

"No. 349: redness of the face, as in scarlatina. 408 to 413: tongue very painful, the burning and raw feeling increases; vesicles spring up along the margin of the tongue, the pains are accompanied by stitches; at the tip of the tongue, toward the left side, a row of small vesicles spring up, some six or eight, which are very painful and sore; dryness of the tongue, red and fiery appearance of the inside of the cheeks, with painful sensitiveness. 311: pains in the interior of the right ear. 413 to 417: burning at the upper portion of the left ear; stitches under the left ear, tension under and behind the ears; red swelling of both ears, with a stinging and burning pain in the swelling. 462 to 463: difficulty of swallowing, staging pains when swallowing. 466: burning in the fauces down to the stomach. 470: difficulty of swallowing in consequence of redness and swelling of the tonsils. 473: ulcers in the throat during scarlet fever. 1236: scarlatina does not come out, in the place of which the throat becomes ulcerated. 1237: retrocession of scarlatina, violent fever, excessive heat, congestion of the head, reddened eyes, violent delirium. 832: redness and swelling in front of the neck, swelling of the glands. 833: swelling of the cervical glands on the injured side. 836: tension on the right side of the nape of the neck, below and back of the ear. 897, 898: itching and burning of the dorsum of the hand and [38] of the knuckles and first phalanges; cracking of the skin here and there; itching and chapping of the hand and lower lip."

If we add to these symptoms the above enumerated cerebral symptoms, the typhoid alteration of the internal mucous membrane of the whole alimentary canal and of the respiratory organs, the disorganizing and paralyzing action upon the blood and nerves, the inclination to dropsical effusion, the affection of the cervical glands with tendency to suppuration, the appearance of otorrhœa,—we have a group of symptoms which resemble very accurately the prevailing type of epidemic scarlatina. I know, from abundant experience, that the homœopathic law has been brilliantly confirmed in this disease. Thanks to the curative powers of Apis, scarlatina has ceased to be a scourge to childhood. The dangers to which children were usually exposed in scarlatina, have dwindled down to one, which fortunately is a comparatively rare phenomenon. It is only where the scarlet-fever poison acts at the outset with so much intensity, that the brain becomes paralyzed at once, and the disease must necessarily terminate fatally, that no remedy has as yet been discovered. In all other cases, unless some strange mishap should interfere, the physician, who is familiar with Apis, need not fear any untoward results in his treatment of scarlatina.

In all lighter cases, where the disease sets in less tumultuously, and runs a mild course, it is proper, as soon as the disease has fairly broken out, to give a globule of Apis 30, and to watch the effects of this [39] dose without interference. The immediate consequence of this proceeding, is to bring the eruption out in a few hours, all over the skin, with abatement of the fever and general perspiration, after which the eruption runs its course in a few days, with a progressive feeling of convalescence, the epidermis peels off from the third to the fifth day, and, at the latest, to the seventh day, with cessation of the fever, so that the process of desquamation is generally terminated within the next seven days, after *which the patient may be fairly said to be convalescent, and the patient may be said to be absolutely freed from all danger of consecutive diseases.*

The same result is obtained by nature in cases of mild scarlatina, without the interference of art. But the experience which I have had an opportunity of making during my long official employment as district-physician, has convinced me that Nature accomplishes her end far more easily, more speedily and satisfactorily, if assisted by art in accordance with the law of homœopathy. The sequelæ especially are rendered less dangerous by this means.

But if the disease sets in with a considerable degree of intensity at the very outset, and the fever continues without abatement, it is advisable to keep up a medicinal impression by repeating the dose. To this end we dissolve a globule of Apis 30, in seven dessert-spoonfuls of water, by shaking the solution vigorously in a corked vial, and giving a dessert-spoonful every three, six, or twelve hours as the case may require. In all ordinary cases a single solution of this kind sufficed to subdue the [40] fever and to secure a favorable termination of the disease.

The struggle between disease and medicine assumes a far different form, if the morbific poison has penetrated the organism more deeply; if a process of disorganization has already developed itself in the intestinal mucous membrane, and if the alteration of the sanguineous fluid, which is an inherent accompaniment of such a disorganizing process, has depressed the nervous activity to such a degree that typhus, or paralysis of the brain or lungs seems unavoidable, as may be inferred from the bright-red tongue, which is thickly studded with eruptive vesicles, and speedily becomes excoriated, fissured and covered with aphthæ; by a copious discharge of thick, white, bloody and fetid mucus from the nose; by the swelling and induration of the parotid glands, increasing difficulty of deglutition; sensitiveness of the abdomen to pressure; badly-colored, slimy, bloody diarrhœa; scanty emissions of turbid, red, painful urine; accelerated and labored breathing; loss of consciousness; delirium; sopor; convulsions; trembling of the limbs; appearance as if the patient were lying in his bed in a state of fainting; the skin is at times burning, hot and dry; at others it feels like parchment, cooler; at others again, hot and cool together in spots; the fever increases with changing pulse, and is more constant; in short, all the symptoms, although developing themselves less rapidly, show that a fatal termination becomes more and more probable. In such a case it is above all things [41] necessary to saturate the organism with Apis. If there is much fever, this result is best accomplished by means of alternate doses of Aconite and Apis, a few drops of the third potency, shaken together with twelve tablespoonfuls of water, each drug by itself, the dose to be repeated every hour; and if the temperature is rather depressed, by giving Apis without the Aconite, a tablespoonful every hour or two hours. In favorable cases the fever becomes more remittent within one to three days; a moderate and pleasant perspiration breaks out all over the skin; the sleep becomes calm and natural, and the typhoid symptoms abate. If this change takes place, it is proper to exhibit Apis in a more dynamic form, in order to assimilate it more harmoniously to the newly awakened reactive power of the organism. To this end we dissolve a few globules of Apis 30 in seven dessert-spoonfuls of water, giving a dessert-spoonful morning and evening, and we continue this treatment, until the symptoms of typhoid angina have gradually abated, the tongue has been healed, the normal desire for food has returned, and the digestive functions go on regularly; after which the natural reaction of the organism, assisted by careful diet, will be found sufficient to complete the cure. If no improvement sets in after Apis has been used for three days, we may rest assured that a psoric miasm is in the way of a cure, which requires to be combated with some anti-psoric remedy. I have generally found Kali carbonicum efficient, of which I gave one globule thirty on the fourth day of the treatment, permitting [42] it to act uninterruptedly from one to three days, according as the disease was more or less acute, after which I again exhibited Apis in the manner previously indicated. In this way I succeeded in developing the curative powers of Apis, so that in a few days a gradual improvement, however slight, became perceptible to the careful observer. As soon as the improvement is well marked, all repetition of the medicine should cease, and the natural reaction of the organism should be permitted to complete the cure. Any one who is acquainted with the action of the Kali, must know that it continues without being interrupted by Apis. An invaluable blessing of Nature!

This proceeding is crowned with the desired results; the convalescence is shorter and easier, and there is less danger of serious sequelæ, which, according to all experience, are so common in complicated cases of scarlatina, otorrhœa and suppuration of the parotid glands are generally avoided under this treatment without any other aid, or, if it is impossible to avert such changes, they generally come to a speedy and safe end. This treatment likewise keeps off dropsy and its dangers.

In cases where the secretion of *black urine* shows that the liver is deeply involved in the disease, Apis is powerless. These are the only exceptions to the curative power of this drug. Here we are told by our law of cure, that the sphere of Lachesis commences. We give one or two globules of Lachesis 30 in seven dessert-spoonfuls of water, a dessert-spoonful [43] every twelve hours, and in acute cases every three hours; and the good effects of the medicine must seem miraculous to one who is not accustomed to this mode of treating diseases. Already in a few hours the patient becomes tranquil, showing that the process of disorganization has been arrested; the improvement continues from hour to hour; the sleep becomes more tranquil; the cutaneous secretions, and those of the bowels and kidneys, become more active; after the lapse of one, or at most two days, the urine begins to look clearer and lighter-colored, and in about three days a return of the natural color of the urine shows that the functions of the liver are restored to their normal standard; the patient is able to do without any further medical treatment, and the natural reaction of the vital forces will be found sufficient to effect a cure.

If I have not mentioned the affections of the kidneys, which may be present in this disease, it is because I have become satisfied by years of experience, that they constitute secondary affections in scarlatina, and that we should commit a great error if we would draw conclusions regarding this point from post-mortem phenomena.

Nobody who has observed the resemblance, at any rate, during the present epidemic, between

RUBEOLA

and scarlet-fever, will deny that the remarks which [44] we have offered concerning this latter disease, likewise apply to rubeola. In

MEASLES,

likewise, Apis will prove a curative agent.

In the American Provings, Apis is indicated in this disease by the following symptoms: "No. 1103, heat all over; the face is red as in scarlatina; eruption like measles; cough and difficult respiration as in croup; muttering delirium; 1211, superficial eruptions over the whole body, resembling measles, with great heat and a reddish-blue circumscribed flush on the cheeks; 1218, measle-shaped eruption."

If we add to these symptoms the peculiarity inherent in Apis, to cause catarrhal irritations of the eyes, such as occur during measles, we have a right to infer that Apis will prove a valuable remedial agent in measles.

Although common mild measles do not require any medicinal treatment, and generally get well without any prejudice to the general health; nevertheless, cases occur where intense ophthalmia, a violent and racking cough, and the phenomena which appertain to it; an intense irritation of the internal mucous membrane; diarrhœa; dangerous prostration of strength; marked stupefaction and various nervous phenomena render the interference of art desirable. In all such cases, I have seen good effects from the use of Apis, which differed not only from the regular course of the disease, but likewise from the effects which have been witnessed [45] under the operation of other medicines. In ordinary cases, and without treatment, it takes three, five, seven and eleven days, before the eyes get well again; but under the use of Apis, the eyes improve so decidedly in from one to three days, that the eyes do not require any further treatment; and that even troublesome sequelæ, such as photophobia; styes which come and go; troublesome lachrymation; continual redness; swelling and blennorrhœa of the lids; fistulæ lachrymalis, etc., need not be apprehended.

If Apis has had a chance to exercise its curative action in a case of measles, we hear nothing of the troublesome, and often so wearing and racking cough, which so often prevails in measles, and the continuance of which is accompanied by an increased irritation and swelling of the respiratory mucous membrane and an increasing alteration of its secretion, which recurs in paroxysms, assumes a suspicious sound, shows a tendency to croup and to the development of tuberculosis, and finally degenerates in whooping-cough, so that epidemic measles and whooping-cough often go hand in hand. After Apis, the cough speedily begins to become looser and milder, to loose its dubious character, and to gradually disappear without leaving a trace behind. If these results should be confirmed by further experience, we would have attained additional means of preventing the supervention of whooping-cough in measles; a triumph of art and science which should elicit our warmest gratitude.

Any one who knows, how malignant measles, [46] unassisted by art, are accompanied by deep-seated irritation of the mucous membrane of the stomach and bowels; how they lead to diarrhœa; to sopor; how they threaten life by long-lasting and troublesome putrid and typhoid fevers; and how, if they do not terminate fatally, they result in slow convalescence, and sometimes in chronic maladies for life, will admit, on seeing the diarrhœa cease; on beholding the quiet sleep which patients enjoy; the pleasant and general perspiration; the return of appetite; the increase of strength, and the complete disappearance of all putrid and typhoid symptoms, that Apis has indeed triumphed over the disease.

The following simple proceeding will secure such results: As soon as the fever has commenced, we prepare the above-mentioned solution of Aconite, of which we give a small spoonful every hour. If, after using the Aconite, the eruption breaks out and the fever abates, no further medication is necessary. If fever and eruption should require further aid, Apis is to be given, one or two globules of thirtieth potency in seven dessert-spoonfuls of water, well shaken, a dessert-spoonful morning and evening; or, if the disease is very acute, every three hours, which treatment is to be continued until an improvement sets in, after which the natural reaction of the organism will terminate the cure.

Sequelæ seldom take place after this kind of treatment; this is undoubtedly an additional recommendation for the use of Apis. Until this day I have never seen a secondary disease resulting from measles. Nevertheless, such sequelæ will [47] undoubtedly occur, for it is characteristic of the measle-miasm, to rouse latent psoric, sycosic, syphilitic and vaccinine taints, which afterwards require a specific anti-psoric treatment. Nevertheless, sequelæ will certainly occur less frequently after the use of Apis, for which we ought to be thankful. In

URTICARIA AND PEMPHIGUS

Apis will likewise afford speedy and certain help.

Many symptoms in the American Provings confirm this statement. More particularly 1198 to 1210, and 1232 to 35: "very soon thick nettle-rash over the whole body, itching a good deal, passing off after sleeping soundly; violent inflammation and pressure over the whole body; friction brought out small white spots resembling musquito-bites; suddenly an indescribable stinging sensation over the whole body, with white and red spots in the palms of the hands, on the arms and feet; her Whole body was covered with itching and burning swollen streaks, after which the other troubles disappeared; swelling of the face and body; the parts are covered with a sort of blotches somewhat paler than the ordinary color of the skin; eruption over the whole body resembling nettle-rash, with itching and burning; nettle-rash in many cases; spots on the nape of the neck and forehead, resembling nettle-rash under the skin; consequences of repelled urticaria; whitish, violently itching swellings of the skin, on the head and nape of the neck, like nettle-rash; [48] after the rash disappeared, the whole of the right side was paralyzed, with violent delirium even unto rage; after taking Apis the eruption appeared in abundance, and the delirium abated."

These provings have been abundantly confirmed by my own experience. The use of Apis in these eruptions has been followed in my hands by the most satisfactory results; and I feel justified in recommending Apis as a most efficient remedy in these diseases, which are still wrapt in a good deal of obscurity. An additional source of satisfaction to have obtained more means of relieving human suffering. The experienced Neuman writes, in his Special Therapeutics, 2d Edit., Vol. I., Section 2, p. 681, about urticaria: "Howsoever unimportant a single eruption of urticaria may be, it becomes disagreeable and troublesome by its constant repetition, which is not dangerous, but exceedingly disturbing. It would be desirable to be acquainted with a safe method of curing this eruption, but so far, it has been sought for in vain." The same physician, speaking of pemphigus, writes in the same place, that its etiology, prognosis and treatment, are still very dubious; that it leads to extensive chronic sufferings, and often terminates fatally; and that no specific remedy is known for this disease. The more frequent opportunities we have of observing both these diseases in different individuals, the more frequently we observe them in conjunction with serious chronic maladies characterized by some specific chronic miasm, or in conjunction with the most penetrating and disturbing emotions, such as [49] fright and its consequences; the more frequently we observe the sudden appearance and disappearance of such pustules, alternating with corresponding improvements or exacerbations in the internal organism, where we have to look on utterly powerless, as it were, the more uneasy do we feel at the mysterious nature of this malady, which, during the period of organic vigor, seems to be a sort of trifling derangement, somewhat like urticaria, but which, as the vital energies become prostrated by age, becomes more and more searching and tormenting, breaks forth again and again, exhausting the vital juices and leading irresistibly to a fatal termination; a result which is particularly apt to take place during old age, although I have likewise observed it, but rarely, among new-born infants.

These developments lead us to suspect that urticaria and pemphigus are identical in essence; this fact is richly substantiated by the homœopathic law which furnishes identical means of cure for either of these affections. In either case, if the vital forces are prostrated, and the sensitiveness of the organic reaction is considerable, one pellet of Apis 30, and, if there is considerable resistance to overcome, two pellets shaken with six dessert-spoonfuls of water, a spoonful night and morning, is all that should be done, after which, all further treatment should be discontinued as long as the improvement continues or the skin remains clear from all eruptions. If the improvement cease or the eruption should reappear, we have in the first place to examine whether the improvement will not speedily resume [50] its course, or whether the eruption does not show itself more feebly than before, or if the cure is not evidenced by some other favorable change. In the former case the medicine should be permitted to act still further; in the latter case, another dose of Apis 30 should be given, after which the result has to be carefully watched. In all benign cases, more particularly if no other means of treatment had been resorted to before, this management will suffice. If this should not be the case, if the eruption should appear again, we may rest assured that a psoric miasm lurks in the organism, and that an anti-psoric treatment has to be resorted to. The best anti-psoric under these circumstances, is Sulphur 30, one pellet, provided this drug has not yet been abused; or Causticum 30, one pellet, if such an abuse has taken place. Syphilis may likewise complicate the disease, in which case Mercurius 30, one pellet, may be given; or, if Mercury had been previously taken in excessive doses, Mercurius 6000, one globule.

After one or the other of these remedies, the symptoms should be carefully observed without doing anything else, with a view of instituting whatever treatment may afterwards be necessary, we wind up the treatment with another dose of Apis 30, one pellet, after which, the organic power is permitted to complete the cure. The result is, that the most difficult and complicated cases yield perfectly to such treatment, which is based upon the strictest scientific principles. [51]

FURUNCLES AND CARBUNCLES

are likewise cured by Apis in the speediest and easiest manner.

We find the following symptomatic indications in the American Provings: "682, painful pimple, suppurating in the middle, with red areola; painful like a boil, in the hairy region on the left side above the os pubis, continuing painful for several days; 1196, furuncles with stinging pains; 844, 845, violent, stinging, burning pain at a small spot on the left side, in the lower region of the nape of the neck; also on the back part of the head; swelling at the nape of the neck, so that the head is pressed forward towards the chest; 1222, dark bluish-red painful swellings, with general malaise; 1167, acute pain and erysipelatous swelling, very hard and pale in the centre."

Apis has been a popular remedy for boils from time immemorial; the people have been in the habit of covering boils with honey, more particularly honey in which a bee had perished.

Apis, homœopathically prepared, is better adapted to such an end than honey. A few drops of Apis 3, shaken with twelve tablespoonfuls of water, a tablespoonful of this solution every three hours, generally relieves the pain in a short period, promotes suppuration, effects the discharge of the decayed cellular tissue, and a speedy cure of the furuncle.

If furuncles incline to become carbunculous, the [52] ichorous matter is speedily changed to good pus, and all danger is averted.

In a case of carbuncle the gangrenous disorganization of the skin and cellular tissue becomes very soon confined to a small spot; the dead parts are separated from the living tissues; the fever is hushed; the disorganizations which it threatens are averted; a healthy suppuration is established throughout the gangrenous part, detaching and removing all decayed matter, and replacing the loss of substance by new granulations until the sore becomes cicatrized in such a hardly perceptible manner, that any one who is acquainted with the ravages of this disease, and is in the habit of seeing deep and disfiguring cicatrizes, even in the most successful cases, is disposed to deny the fact that such an intensely disorganizing process has been going on in this instance. No other remedial means are required, much less a surgical operation.

Inasmuch as carbuncle is generally preceded for a longer period by a deep-seated feeling of illness in the organism, showing that the psoric miasm pervades the tissues, it behooves us, in order to secure all the better a favorable result, to give a dose of highly-potentized Sulphur at the very outset of the disease. After having used the first portion of Apis, a globule of Sulphur 30 or 6000 may be interposed, the former in all cases where no Sulphur had been used, and the latter in cases Sulphur had been used in large doses. We permit such a dose to act for twenty-four hours, after which [53] Apis is resumed, and continued according to the above stated rule.

Sulphur should likewise be given in all cases where the furuncles reappear at different periods. Such a reappearance of the eruption, after it had once been cured by Apis, shows that a psoric taint pervades the organism which it is absolutely necessary to meet with specific counter-acting remedies.

The more frequently we meet such difficult complications, and see with our own eyes their successful treatment, the more we learn to appreciate the fact, *that Apis cures to a certainty the most dangerous affections of this kind, and that the anti-psoric remedy corrects at the same time the primary degeneration of the tissues, without either interfering with the operations of the other drug, on the contrary, by assisting each other.* In

PANARITIA

Apis proves the same invaluable remedy.

Genuine panaritia only spring up in psoric ground, and in regard to extent and intensity of development, depend altogether upon the existing psoric taint. Hence it is indispensable to extinguish this taint by appropriate remedies. This is most effectually accomplished by at once giving Sulphur, the most powerful of our anti-psorics. Sulphur seems to attack the evil at its very foundation, and we feel perfectly satisfied with its action, except that we would like to hasten the course of the disease still more, in order to abbreviate the [54] tortures inherent in this malady. This result is most certainly accomplished by means of Apis.

If panaritia are the result of excessive doses of Sulphur, Apis meets our case perfectly. In hundreds of cases panaritia spring up and will continue to spring up from such a source, as long as the world continues to live in darkness, and to reject the rays of truth which the genius of Hahnemann has sent forth among the benighted understandings of his fellow beings. Notwithstanding Hahnemann's teachings concerning the medicinal power of Sulphur, which the world has now been in possession of for years, and which the most thoughtful minds have accepted as a truth, the true friend of man has still to weep over the quantities of Sulphur which all apothecaries sell to any one at his option; hæmorrhoidal patients continue to swallow Sulphur from day to day; almost every body, from the child up to the old man, who is affected with catarrh, swallows the so-termed pulmonary powders which contain Sulphur, and of which relief is expected; whole legions repair every year to the Sulphur Springs; young and old use sulphur-baths at home; all over the world, the itch, which is a very common disease, is removed by means of a sulphur ointment, &c. One of the evil consequences of this ignorance, which particularly oppresses the laboring class, is the artificial development of panaritia; the more frequently these occur, the more necessary it is to employ speedy and safe means for their extermination. In such a case we can no longer depend upon Sulphur, of which we cannot possibly know [55] how far it has already poisoned the organism, and to what extent it may still be able to rouse a reaction; in which case, even those who know, may be led to make dangerous mistakes. In all such cases Apis is of the best use to us; it is even sufficient to arrest the disorganizing process, and to bring about a satisfactorily progressing cure.

The curative indications contained in the "American Provings," have been confirmed by my own experience. We read in Nos. 903-911, "the phalangeal bones are painful; burning jerking, like a stitching, contracting sensation, in the right numb, from without inwards; drawing pains reaching the extremities of the fingers; distinct feeling of numbness in the fingers, especially in the tips, around the roots of the nails, with sensation as if the nails were loose, and as if they could be shaken off; burning in the tips of fingers, as from fire; fine burning stinging in the tips of the fingers; burning around a hang-nail, on the outside of the fourth finger of the right hand, with pain internally, without redness and without aggravation from pressure, with continual burning in the tip; swelling of the fingers, which remained painful for several days; 915, blister at the tip of the right index, discharging a bloody ichor when opened, and afterwards a milky pus, with violent burning, throbbing, and gnawing pains, continuing to spread for two days."

From all this we deduce the highly important practical rule: In a case of whitlow, first ascertain whether and how far Sulphur has been abused by the patient. Unfortunately the non-abuse of Sulphur [56] is an exception to the rule, whereas the abuse of Sulphur is quite common even in our age. Would that in this respect the ancient darkness might yield to the new light.

In case Sulphur had been abused by the patient, we mix a few drops of Apis 3 in twelve tablespoonfuls of water, giving a tablespoonful every hour, or every two or three hours, according as the pains are more or less violent. This treatment has to be continued until the pains cease. They cease either because the inflammation has been dispersed, and the morbid process is terminated, or else a healthy suppuration has been set up, so that the swelling will discharge of itself, and a cure will be effected as speedily as the nature of the panaritium will admit. In either case the medicine need not be repeated, and the organic reaction will be sufficient to complete a cure without the interference of surgery. A simple bread and milk poultice may be used as soothing palliative, especially if the external skin is of a firm, hard texture. Resolution may be depended upon in every case, where Apis has been resorted to in time. A healthy suppuration will always set in after the exhibition of Apis, provided Sulphur or a psoric taint do not gain the ascendancy. If the Sulphur miasm gains the ascendancy, there will be no marked improvement during the first days of the treatment. In such a case we have at once to resort to a very high potency of Sulphur. A single globule of Sulphur 6000 would frequently ameliorate the worst aspect of the case as by a miracle, after which a few more doses of Apis 3, a [57] drop morning and evening, would so improve the symptoms, as to render all further medication unnecessary.

If the psoric miasm should be the cause of the retarded improvement, as may easily be determined by the predisposing circumstances of the case, and if no Sulphur should have been administered previously, it is expedient to discontinue the use of Apis, and to at once exhibit a globule of Sulphur 30, which may be allowed to act for twenty-four hours, after which Apis is to be resumed in the same manner, until a cessation of the pain manifests the cure of the disease.

These explanations likewise point out the true course to be pursued, in case we should at the outset find that a whitlow owes its existence to the psoric miasm.

Ever since homœopathy has enabled us to treat this dreaded affection with positive and specific remedies in a most satisfactory manner, the horrible pains which characterize this trouble, and the mutilations to which it so frequently leads, only exist in quarters where egotism, the love of lucre and the absence of all conscientiousness prevents physicians from inquiring into the merits of our superior mode of treatment. Is not this unpardonably wicked?

SPONTANEOUS LIMPING

is another affection which we cure with Apis.

This disease which causes so much distress in life, is likewise, in its essential nature, an outbirth [58] of psora, and, as regards its local character and its effects upon the constitution of the patient, it seems to be characterized by the same inflammatory and suppurative process as whitlow, and be endowed with a similar tendency to organic destruction. In the American Provings, symptom 917, "Painful soreness in the left hip-joint, immediately after taking a dose of Apis 2, afterwards debility, unsteadiness, trembling in this joint," is the only symptom that seems to indicate the curative power of Apis in this distressing malady. What experienced physician has not often seen the hip show such symptoms of disease, particularly after violent frights and anguish? Who has not seen blows on the back and nates, by way of punishment, attended with such consequences? Who has not seen coxarthrocace develop itself during the course of a severe cerebral disease, scarlatina or typhus, where the patient, on suddenly awakening to consciousness from a state of stupor, is made sensitive of the presence of this insidious disease, perhaps already fully developed? Since I have used Apis, I have never had to deplore such saddening results.

According to my observation, we may regard Apis as a specific remedy for spontaneous limping; every new trial confirms me in this statement. Apis may be depended upon as a capital remedy in every stage of this disease, as long as the psoric miasm is kept in the background; but as soon as the psoric taint is fully developed, a suitable anti-psoric has to be given in alternation with Apis. My experience has led me to prefer Kali carbonicum [59] to all other anti-psoric remedies in this disease. But inasmuch as the keenest observer may overlook the right moment when the psoric poison begins to operate, it is well to forestall the enemy at the very commencement, which may be done with the more propriety, the more certainly we know that these two remedies, Apis and the anti-psoric, not only not counteract, but mutually support each other from the beginning to the end of the treatment. After many experiments, I have hit upon the following course as the most proper:

If the limping, as is often the case in the severest forms of the disease, sets in gradually, almost imperceptibly and without much pain, I give at once a globule of Kali carbonicum 30. As a general rule, this one dose is sufficient to arrest the further development of the disease, and to award all danger so completely, that one, who is unacquainted with the nature of the malady, feels disposed to assert that it never existed. But if the pains continue, and are accompanied with fever, I resort to Apis 3, after Kali had been allowed to act for a day or two, mixing a drop in twelve tablespoonfuls of water, and giving a dose every hour, or every two or three hours, according as the pains come on more or less frequently. This treatment is continued until the patient is quieted, after which the two remedies are permitted to act without any further repetition of the medicine.

If the inflammation of the joint sets in suddenly and with a violent fever, as is often the case after violent commotions, castigations, etc., we prepare a [60] solution of Aconite in the same manner as the Apis, and give these two medicines in alternate tablespoonful doses every hour. After these two solutions are finished, and the first assault of the disease has been controlled, we give a globule of Kali 30, and permit it to act for twenty-four hours. After this period we again give Apis every hour, two or three hours, as above, until the pains cease, after which Kali is allowed to act until the disease is entirely cured.

If suppuration and caries of the joint have already set in, no matter whether the pus has found an outlet in the region of the joint itself, or burrows down the thigh to find an outlet somewhere else, Kali is no longer sufficient, Silicea has to be exhibited; it is more homœopathic to caries than other anti-psorics. We give a globule of Silicea 30, and allow it to act for two or three days, after which a drop of Apis 3, is repeated morning and night, until the pains — which may require a more frequent exhibition of the drug — cease, and a healthy pus is secreted. After this change is accomplished, Silicea is sufficient to complete the healing of the osseous disorganization, and should be left undisturbed to the end of the treatment.

I have found this simple proceeding so perfectly efficient in this dreadful malady that the fever was speedily controlled, and rendered harmless, the inflammation was scattered without leaving a trace behind, the secretion ichor was transformed into that of healthy pus, and the disorganization of the joint was prevented; the limb, even after it had [61] become elongated, again assumed its normal shape, the carious masses were expelled, the various channels of suppuration were stopped, and the danger of a fatal consumptive fever was averted. If our aid is not sought until *the head of the femur is destroyed, and the bone has completely slipt out of its socket*, it is impossible to prevent shortening and stiffness of the limb. Another splendid triumph over a dreadful source of danger and disease!

WHITE SWELLING OF THE KNEE

is very similar to this affection of the hip-joint. Here too we observe the same insidious inflammatory beginning, the same irresistible tendency to ichorous suppuration and disorganization of the constituent parts of the joint, the same tendency to destroy the organism by gradual exhausting fever. We have unmistakeable proofs of the presence of a poisonous process pervading the whole organism. He who has had frequent opportunities of observing this disease, knows perfectly in what mysterious obscurity it is still enveloped, and how specifically different this affection of the knee sometimes appears to us from the hip disease. The homœopathic law teaches us more positively than any thing else could do, that every case of disease should be viewed as something specifically distinct from other cases, and should be treated with medicines that are specifically adapted to it. An experience of many years has taught me that iodine is the best [62] remedy to meet the symptoms which generally characterize white swelling of the knee. Even at the present day Iodine is one of those remedies that require a good deal of elucidation. Hence we should not, carried away by analogy, conclude from those things which are not clear, concerning other things which are no more so. Nevertheless the observations which have been made so far, have led to some highly important, more or less positive conclusions, and have shown us with a certain degree of satisfaction and certainty, that iodine is an inestimable gift of God, by means of which we are enabled to free mankind from one of the most frightful complications, the psoric, sycosic and mercurial miasms. I have been induced by various signs to believe that, in white swelling of the knee such a complication exists.

Considering the paucity of our observations bearing upon this important point, it seems impracticable to make any positive statements with reference to the assistance that we might possibly derive from the use of Apis in this disease. My own opportunities for observation having been very few, I recommend the use of Apis in white swelling of the knee, to my professional brethren. The following symptoms in "Hering's American Provings," seem to indicate it; No.'s 828, 829 and 931, "violent pain in the left knee, externally, above and below the knee, particularly above, somewhat in front;

painful œdematous swelling of the knee; burning stinging about the knee." In white swelling of the knee, where no allœopathic treatment [63] has yet been pursued, I recommend Iodine 30, one globule, in six dessert-spoonfuls of water, a dessert-spoonful morning and evening, until the whole is finished; after this wait three days, and then give Apis 3, as before mentioned, a tablespoonful every hour or three hours, or a drop morning and evening, according as the pain or danger is more or less pressing. Apis is more especially useful in removing pain, in changing the secretion of ichor to that of healthy pus, and in arresting the consumptive fever. After these results have been accomplished, we permit the previously given Iodine to achieve the cure. If Iodine had been abused under allœopathic treatment, before the homœopathic treatment commenced, we give Iodine 5000, one globule, in order to subdue the Iodine diathesis, and thus remove the most powerful obstacle to a cure. Any one who knows more about this point, will please mention it.

Although Apis acts well in white swelling of the knee, which is comparatively a rare disease, yet it is far more useful in

DYSENTERY.

It is undoubtedly true that Hahnemann has revealed to us the means of surpassing in this disease the allœopathic wisdom of a thousand years, by a far more successful, safe and expeditious treatment. Nevertheless, much remains to be desired in this dreaded disease. Who does not know that medicinal [64] aggravations are particularly to be dreaded in this malady? Who has not often felt embarrassed to select the right remedy among three or four that seemed indicated by the symptoms, and where it was nevertheless important, in view of the threatening danger, to select at once the right remedy? Who has not been struck by the strange irregularity that in a disease which generally sets in as an epidemic, different remedies are often indicated by different groups of symptoms? Who has not become convinced after a careful observation of the course of the disease, that nothing is more deceptive than the pretended curative virtues of corrosive sublimate in dysentery, and that it is a matter of duty to be mindful, in this very particular, of the warning words of the master who, having himself been deceived at one time by the delusive palliation of mercury, addresses to us the remarkable warning that "mercury, so far from responding to all non-venereal maladies, on the contrary is one of the most deceitful palliatives the temporary action of which is not only soon followed by a return of the original symptoms of disease, but even by a return of these symptoms in an aggravated form." (See Hahnemann's Chronic Diseases, Vol. II.)

This delusive palliation is more particularly one of the effects of corrosive sublimate in Dysentery; and is exceedingly dangerous in this disease. Hence we warn practitioners against this danger.

We feel so much the more grateful to the principle Similia Similibus, which, even though it did not protect its discoverer from faulty applications, [65] yet finally led us to the discovery of the right remedy for dysentery.

No.'s 590 and 599 in the American Provings, read as follows: "Violent tenesmus; nausea, vomiting and diarrhœa, first lumpy and not fetid, afterwards watery and fetid, lastly papescent, mixed with blood and mucus, and attended with tenesmus; afterwards dysenteric stools, with tenesmus and sensation as if the bowels were crushed;" combining these symptoms with the general character of Apis, particularly the circumstance that not only the ordinary precursors and first symptoms of dysentery, but also its terminations and its sequelæ, and its most important complications find their approved remedy in Apis; all this shows us that Apis is a natural remedy for dysentery. This truth is abundantly confirmed by experience. All my previously obtained results in practice, testify to the correctness of this statement.

At the very commencement of the disease, a globule of Apis 3 is sufficient to cut short the disease so that the patient feels easy, and sleeps quietly. During this slumber, fever, pain and tenesmus disappear, and the patient wakes with a feeling of health. If this should not take place in three hours, owing to the more advanced state of the disease, another dose of Apis is required, after which the patient soon feels well.

If the dysenteric disease has had a chance to localize itself, and to assume a higher degree of intensity, it becomes necessary to excite the organic reaction all the more frequently. Under these circumstances [66] we repeat the medicine every hour, or every two or three hours, one globule at a time, until all further medication has become unnecessary.

It is well known that epidemic diarrhœa, viz., a diarrhœa resulting from peculiar alterations of the normal condition of the atmosphere, earth, water, indispensable food, or from other still unknown elementary influences inevitably acting upon every body, commences in the form of a simple, apparently unimportant diarrhœa; that it gradually increases in intensity as the processes of nutrition and sanguification become more deeply disturbed, and that it finally terminates in life-destroying cholera. All these different stages of diarrhœa, whether with or without vomiting, watery or papescent, of one color or another, with or without pain, with or without fever, have yielded readily, safely and thoroughly to Apis in my hands. I must except, however, cholera of the epidemic form, where I have not yet been able to try Apis for want of opportunity. As far as my personal observations go, I am disposed to affirm that the best mode of effecting a good result, is to give Apis 3 and Aconite 3, in alternation, one drop of each preparation well shaken in a bottle containing twelve tablespoonfuls of water, and giving a tablespoonful every hour or three hours, if the danger is great, and in milder cases a full drop alternately morning and evening. This treatment is continued until an improvement sets in, after which the organic reaction is permitted to develop itself, which will terminate in a few [67] hours or days, according as the disease is more or less violent, and assistance was sought more or less early, in the perfect recovery of the patient.

This end is not always attained with equal certainty and rapidity, if Apis is not given in alternation with Aconite. In such a case, Apis alone often develops a powerful reaction, which is avoided by the alternate use of Aconite. Wherever the case is urgent, and it is important to shorten the durations of the organic reaction, the two remedies should be given in alternation. In most cases I have seen a few alternate doses give rise to a pleasant perspiration, speedily followed by quiet sleep and recovery on waking. May we not expect the same result at the commencement of Asiatic cholera, and thus arrest the further development of the disease?

Apis is no less effectual against *chronic diarrhœa*, more particularly if resulting, not from any deep-seated disorganizations, but from some permanent inflammatory irritation of the intestinal mucous membrane, and which causes and fosters so much distress, by rendering all normal digestion impossible and finally bringing on its inseparable companion, the last degree of hypochondria. This misery is so much more lamentable, as it is, so to say, forced upon mankind from the cradle to the grave by the still prevailing and almost ineradicable delusion of *cathartic medication*.

Scarcely has the little being seen the light of the world, when the process of purgation begins. Nurse, aunt, grandmamma, everybody, hasten to hush the cries which the rough contact of the outer world [68] extorts from the little being, by forcing down its throat a little laxative mixture, and the family-physician, who goes by fashion, approves of all this. It is his habit, in after-life, to combat every little costiveness, every digestive derangement, every incipient disease, by means of his cathartic mixture, and his skill is considered proportionate to the quantity of stuff which the bowels expel under the operation of his drugs. Laxative pills, rhubarb, glauber-salts, bitter-waters, aloes, gin, etc., etc., are in every body's hands, and become an increasing necessity for millions. An ancient prejudice decrees that, to permit a single day to pass by without stool, would be to expose one's life to the greatest danger. Every year we see thousands rush to warm and cold springs that have the reputation of being possessed with dissolvent and cathartic properties. Those who cannot afford to go to the springs, use artificial mineral water in order to accomplish similar purposes. Very seldom a disease is met with, that is permitted to run its course without dissolvent or cathartic means. It is still a profitable business to sell patent purgatives, such as cider in which a little magnesia has been dissolved.

Everybody feels how offensive these things are to nature; how they attack the stomach and bowels; how they derange digestion and nutrition; how slowly patients recover from the effects of such drugs; how chronic abdominal affections, after having been eased for a while by such drugs, soon return again with redoubled vigor; how the dose has to be increased in order to obtain the same [69] result; how the intervals of relief becomes shorter and shorter, and how, in the end, the stomach is totally ruined, and the abnormal irritation and paralysis of this viscus, with the diarrhœa and constipation, corresponding to these conditions, gradually lead to the complete derangement of the reproductive process.

In spite of all this, long habit has secured to these pernicious customs a sort of prescriptive right. The distress consequent upon them, increases in proportion as the reactive powers of the organism decrease, which is more particularly the case in the present generation. The suppression of these abuses has never been more necessary than in our age. Indeed, the old proverb is again verified: "Where need is greatest, there help is nearest."

The world is not only indebted to Hahnemann for a knowledge, but also for a natural corrective of this serious abuse. His provings on healthy persons show this beyond a doubt. Few men, if their attention has once been directed to this abuse, will feel disposed to deny its extent. Nor has a favorable change in this respect been looked for in vain, since homœopathy has now, for half a century at least, shown the uselessness of all regular methods of purgation, and the superiority of the means with which this new system accomplishes most effectually all that those pernicious methods promised to do. It should be considered a duty by every physician, to be acquainted with the new means of cure. The continued use of purgatives [70] should be considered a crime against health. They will soon cease to exist as regular means of treatment, and their pernicious consequences will no longer have to be relieved by remedial means. But until their use is abolished, we shall have to counteract them by adequate means of cure, more particularly the abnormal irritation and the paralytic debility, which are the most common consequences of the abuse of cathartics.

It is a most fortunate thing that we have in Apis one of the most reliable means of removing the evil effects of cathartic medicines. A single globule of Apis 30 is sufficient to this end. It is best to use it as follows: dissolve the globule in five tablespoonfuls of water by shaking the mixture well in a well closed vial, and let the patient take a tablespoonful of this solution. If this dose acts well, no repetition is necessary for the present. If this dose should not be sufficient, we prepare a new potence by throwing away three tablespoonfuls of the former solution and substituting four tablespoonfuls of fresh water, shaking the mixture well. We give a spoonful of this second solution, twenty-four hours after the first had been given, and, if necessary, a third spoonful prepared in the same way, and even a fourth and fifth, after which we await the result, without thinking either of improvement or exacerbation.

Generally, a feeling of ease is experienced shortly after taking Apis. The painful sensitiveness of the pit of the stomach and of the abdomen, together with the troublesome, disagreeable and oppressive [71] distention and weight, soon disappear; the tongue gradually loses its swollen and cracked appearance, its dirty redness, its slimy coating, its sore spots, tardy indentations along its edges, the burnt feeling at its tip, which is dotted with very fine vesicles, that cause a good deal of soreness; the pappy, sour, bitter, metallic, foul taste disappears; the appetite is again normal; both the previous aversion to food and the excessive craving disappear; the absence of thirst, which is so common in this condition, again gives place to a natural desire for drink, the bluish-red color and swelling of the palate and throat, and the incessant urging to hawk, decrease visibly: the distress after eating; the sour stomach with or without nausea or heartburn; the excessive rising of air; the regurgitation of the ingesta; the eructations which taste of the food that had been eaten long before; the yawning; the irresistible drowsiness when sitting; the general loss of strength; the vacuity of mind, the aversion to talking and to company, decrease more and more every day; the whole abdomen feels easier and softer: the excessive and irresistible urging to urinate, especially after rising from a chair or from bed, and accompanied by a distressing nervousness, abates; the diarrhœic and abnormally colored evacuations, together with the frequent and irresistible urging, increased after eating, early in the morning and after sour and flatulent food, and accompanied by various sore pains in the rectum, diminish more and more, and give place to normal evacuations, first for days, next for weeks, although [72] they continue to alternate more or less with constipation, or painful, insufficient, hard stool, until they terminate sooner or later, according as the disease is more or less deep-seated, and had lasted more or less long, in permanent restoration of the normal secretions and excretions of the digestive organs. At the same time the many distresses which the abnormal condition of the bowels and stomach had occasioned in the head and heart, disappear; the poor patient who had been a prey to so many sufferings, feels like one born again.

This is the general result, unless psoric, sycosic, syphilitic or vaccinine complications should be present. Unfortunately the abuse of cathartics excites these miasms if they exist in the organism, and at the same time prostrates the reactive powers of the organism, and enables its enemies to rise against it. The distress becomes more and more complicated; disorganizations, alterations of the fluids, disturbances of the assimilative sphere, nervous derangements from simple illusions of the sentient sphere, and occasional trembling and twitching, to spasmodic and convulsive movements, and final extinction of nervous power, marasmus of the spinal marrow or a ramollissement of the brain; these are the consequences of such miasmatic complications.

In such a case Apis alone is not sufficient. We have to employ such antidotes as *Sulphur*, our most powerful anti-psoric which, unless it had been abused previously, never leaves us in the lurch in the presence of psora; *iodine* which, under similar circumstances, becomes indispensable wherever psora and [73] sycosis are combined; *bichromate of potash* or *fluoric acid*, if psora, syphilis and mercurial poisoning are united; and lastly, *tartar emetic*, or again *fluoric acid*, if the vaccine poison alone, or in combination with the other poisons, occupies the foreground.

This is not the place to treat of these special forms of human distress, and to individualize their treatment; I shall endeavor to do this on a more suitable occasion. I shall have to limit myself here to a superficial sketch of the treatment, adding merely that a single dose of the specific antidote will act best if given highly potentized, and that the improvement should afterwards be allowed to progress as long as a trace of it remains visible. But as soon as the improvement stops and an exacerbation sets in, which is not speedily followed by another improvement, or which seems to require our aid, we use Apis 3, one drop every day, until the improvement is again perceived, after which we wait until another exacerbation demands our interference. One dose of Apis is often insufficient; if not, from three to five doses will be found sufficient to mitigate the pains, and to advance the cure which Apis will complete in conjunction with the high potency that should not be repeated, and which is not interfered with by the Apis. What more precious boon for the physician and patient in these serious moments? It is only a physician who has instituted provings upon himself, that is capable of comprehending this harmonious blending of the two therapeutic agents. He sees the well known effects of a well known cause go and come at alternate periods. [74] What man of common sense would be willing to repudiate such evidence?

But even in a case where Sulphur and Iodine had been given to excess, and a sort of Sulphur and Iodine diathesis had been established in consequence, Apis is still the best remedy to meet this complicated derangement.

Although we may believe that the time is at hand when this kind of ignorance shall no longer be tolerated, it unfortunately is still a prevailing sin of the profession. Even if we should be unable to effect a perfect cure, yet we may afford essential relief to such patients; we may often arrest their sufferings for a longer or shorter period, and shorten the paroxysms until they become almost imperceptible. Apis is particularly instrumental in effecting this end. Diseases of the

RESPIRATORY ORGANS

are likewise successfully combated by Apis. The American Provings contain the following symptomatic indications:

1. No.'s 731, 733, 736, 742, 743, 749, 760: "Hoarseness and difficulty of breathing, roughness and sensitiveness in the larynx, each time after he smells of the poison; talking is painful, sensation as if the larynx were tired by talking; drawing pains in the larynx; cough when starting during sleep; rough cough during evening; heat; difficult breathing, every drop of liquid almost suffocates him; labored inspirations as during croup." [75]

2. 737-740: "Violent paroxysms of cough, occasioned by a titillating irritation in the lower part of the larynx near the throat-pit, with increase of headache when coughing, on the left side, superiorly; in half an hour, some phlegm is detached, after which the coughing ceases; on the first day, when waked from his sleep before midnight, he had a violent cough, especially after lying down and sleeping, with titillation at a very small spot, deep down on the posterior wall of the thorax, which wakes him; he feels better as soon as the least little portion of mucous is detached; cough particularly during warmth, during rest, and rousing him from his first slumber for several evenings."

3. 1081, 746, 790: "Chilly every afternoon at three or four o'clock; she shudders, especially during warmth; chill across the back, the hands feel as if dead; in about an hour she felt hot and feverish, with rough cough, hot cheeks and hands, without thirst; this passes off gradually, she feels heavy and prostrate; cough and labored breathing as during croup, after violent feverish heat, with dry skin and full pulse; disturbed sleep, with muttering, timid and incoherent talk, whitish-yellow coating of the tongue, and painless, yellow-greenish, slimy diarrhœa, in four days the breathing become labored, a violent abdominal respiration, red face, increasingly livid, pulse hard, cough, with barking resonance—pains in the chest, with labored breathing."

4. 754, 770, 772, 803: "Hurried, labored breathing, with heat and headache; chest oppressed; difficult labored breathing; sense of

suffocation even [76] when leaning against a thing; general debility; worse during cold weather, accompanied by asthmatic pains; cough; sense of suffocation; pains in the chest; coldness and deadness of the extremities, which looked bluish; sense of soreness; lameness; sense of bruising in the chest, as after recent contusions by a blow; jamming, etc."

These observations do not indeed show with characteristic certainty the diseases to which Apis might correspond. But if they are contrasted with the total character of Apis; if we consider that Apis develops a catarrhal irritation throughout the whole intestinal mucous membrane, affecting most deeply the nervous system and the normal constitution of the fluids, we have sufficient ground to experiment with Apis in those respiratory diseases which seem to be inherent in the prevailing genius of disease, and which are characterized by the very conditions which I have described. Who is not struck by the fact, that the same individual morbid process is reflected by different forms of disease, *croup, whooping-cough, influenza, acute and chronic bronchial catarrh*? The more essential the resemblance between these forms of disease and the medicinal power, the more certainly may we expect a cure. The medicinal power which seems to be most adequate to this end, is undoubtedly Apis. My observations in this respect are not sufficiently numerous to enable me to offer positive directions concerning the best mode of using the medicine in these diseases, or concerning the extent of the curative process or the complications that may [77] exist. All I can do is to recommend Apis for further experiments in this range, and to remind my brethren of the insufficiency of other drugs, which has been a source of trouble to us in the past ten years. Every body who has watched the course of these diseases during this period, must have seen the difference existing between the present and the past character of the symptoms. It must, therefore, be a source of satisfaction to all of us, to have found in Apis an agent that is capable of filling up the gap.

My observations regarding the curative virtues of Apis in urinary, uterine and ovarian difficulties, and in rheumatism and gout, are not very extended. In the American Provings, symptoms 634 to 669, seem to point to urinary difficulties, and 685 to 695, to ovarian troubles; symptoms 697 to 727 to uterine derangements; and 837,

842, 867, 873, 874, 918, 919, 940, 942, 964, 969, to rheumatism and gout.

What little experience I have had in the employment of Apis in these diseases, is, however, sufficient to induce me to recommend the use of it for further and more enlarged knowledge.

I have had abundant opportunities of verifying the warning expressed in No. 721, "pregnant women should use the drug very cautiously." I am not acquainted with any drug which seems possessed of such reliable virtues regarding the prevention of miscarriage, more particularly during the first half of pregnancy, as Apis. I have often become an involuntary spectator of the power of Apis to effect miscarriage; for I had given it to honest women [78] who did not know that they were pregnant, and where the fact of pregnancy was revealed to them by the subsequent miscarriage, which took place after one or two doses of Apis had been taken. Ever since I have made it a rule not to give Apis to females in whom the existence of pregnancy can be suspected in the remotest degree until the matter is reduced to a certainty, and the conduct of the physician can be determined upon in accordance with existing facts.

I am unable to say how far this power inherent in Apis, of producing miscarriage, may be serviceable to females who are prone to miscarriage.

I beg the privilege of adding a more general warning to this particular one. The more generally useful a thing is, the more liable is it to abuse. The most important and useful discoveries of homœopathy are abused in this manner by our age given to all sorts of excesses.

Not only are the records of homœopathy ransacked by speculative minds, who use her advantages for personal gain without giving due credit to the source whence the good things are obtained. This species of egotism may perhaps be excused in consideration of the use which this kind of plagiarism affords, even if whole volumes should be filled with it. But if the stolen property is paraded before the world as something belonging to one's self by right divine; if official influence is abused for the purpose of dressing up that which rightfully belongs to our science, as some original discovery, thus caricaturing and disfiguring the beauty of the genuine blessing; [79] then good is changed to evil, and the evil is the greater, the more comprehensive the truth that is so shamefully abused. It is absurd and may entail sad consequences upon the world, if the rational use of Apis is to be converted to the irrational proceedings of the so-called specific method, which is often practised by men who, knowing better, purposely conceal the truth from the world. For years past, I have been called upon again and again, by patients who had been in the hands of these men, and who had been drenched with medicine, and had had all sorts of disastrous complications engendered in their poor bodies, to afford them some relief from these tortures inflicted by physicians who do not hesitate to assail the health of their patients by massive doses of drugs, of which they often know nothing but the name.

With these facts before me, nobody can find it strange that I should feel some misgivings in laying before the world a drug endowed with such extensive virtues. Apis is one of those drugs, the abuse of which may prove as destructive as the use of it is a source of saving good. It is no anti-psoric, nor is it capable of antidoting the three miasms, or of inflicting medicinal diseases for life. Nevertheless, it is a deeply and speedily-acting drug, for it affects the whole internal mucous membrane, the nervous system, and the process of sanguification, thus disturbing the health for a long time. Its primary aggravating action, its deeply penetrating interference with the existing morbid process, which may lead to errors in diagnosis, and its power to [80] exhaust the reactive energies of the organism prematurely, render it a very dangerous agent. These circumstances go to show that such an agent, in the hands of the partizans of the Specific School, may be as dangerously and injuriously abused as other important drugs have been. I cannot sufficiently warn my readers against such distressing abuses. Only he is protected from the danger of imitating such shameful absurdities, who listens to the words of our master:

"Imitate this, but imitate this correctly!"